Cambridge Elements ≡

Elements of Improving Quality and Safety in Healthcare
edited by
Mary Dixon-Woods,* Katrina Brown,* Sonja Marjanovic,†
Tom Ling,† Ellen Perry,* and Graham Martin*
*THIS Institute (The Healthcare Improvement Studies Institute)
†RAND Europe

IMPLEMENTATION SCIENCE

Paul Wilson[1] and Roman Kislov[2]

[1]Centre for Primary Care and Health Services Research, University of Manchester
[2]Centre for Decent Work and Productivity, Manchester Metropolitan University

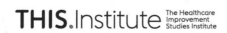 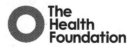

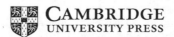

CAMBRIDGE
UNIVERSITY PRESS

University Printing House, Cambridge CB2 8BS, United Kingdom

One Liberty Plaza, 20th Floor, New York, NY 10006, USA

477 Williamstown Road, Port Melbourne, VIC 3207, Australia

314–321, 3rd Floor, Plot 3, Splendor Forum, Jasola District Centre,
New Delhi – 110025, India

103 Penang Road, #05–06/07, Visioncrest Commercial, Singapore 238467

Cambridge University Press is part of the University of Cambridge.

It furthers the University's mission by disseminating knowledge in the pursuit of
education, learning, and research at the highest international levels of excellence.

www.cambridge.org
Information on this title: www.cambridge.org/9781009237086
DOI: 10.1017/9781009237055

First published 2022

A catalogue record for this publication is available from the British Library.

ISBN 978-1-009-23708-6 Paperback
ISSN 2754-2912 (online)
ISSN 2754-2904 (print)

Implementation Science

Elements of Improving Quality and Safety in Healthcare

DOI: 10.1017/9781009237055
First published online: October 2022

Paul Wilson[1] and Roman Kislov[2]
[1]Centre for Primary Care and Health Services Research, University of Manchester
[2]Centre for Decent Work and Productivity, Manchester Metropolitan University

Author for correspondence: Paul Wilson, Paul.Wilson@manchester.ac.uk

Abstract: This Element introduces and critically reflects on the contribution of implementation science to healthcare improvement efforts. Grounded in several disciplines, implementation science is the study of strategies to promote the uptake of evidence-based interventions into healthcare practice and policy. The field's focus is threefold. First, it encompasses theory and empirical research focused on exploring, identifying, and understanding the systems, behaviours, and practices that influence successful implementation. Second, it examines the evaluation of strategies to address barriers or enablers to implementation in a given context. Last, it increasingly seeks to understand the process of implementation itself: what actually gets implemented, and when, why, and how? Despite the growing body of evidence, challenges remain. Many important messages remain buried in the literature, and their impact on implementation efforts in routine practice may be limited. The challenge is not just to get evidence into practice, but also to get implementation science into practice. This title is also available as Open Access on Cambridge Core.

Keywords: implementation science, de-implementation, theory, mechanisms, dissemination

ISBNs: 9781009237086 (PB), 9781009237055 (OC)
ISSNs: 2754-2912 (online), 2754-2904 (print)

Contents

1 Introduction

Establishing the effectiveness of an intervention does not guarantee its adoption into routine practice. Although long recognised, the challenges of getting evidence into practice have become increasingly prominent in recent years as attention has focused on the performance of health systems and the need to ensure that patients benefit from new evidence. Addressing the research–practice gap has spawned a new field that has come to be known as implementation science. Grounded in several disciplines, implementation science is the study of strategies to promote uptake of evidence-based interventions into healthcare practice and policy. The field includes (but is not limited to) the study of professional, patient, and organisational behaviour change. It has championed increased use of empirical research and of theoretical approaches to understand, guide, and evaluate implementation.

In this Element, we describe many of the ideas, theories, and strategies that have emerged from the field over the last decade or so, highlighting how they are or could be applied in practice. We then critically reflect on the overall contribution of the field, outlining a range of challenges in relation to the role and use of theory, the need for mechanism-based explanations of change, and how best to rigorously evaluate change in complex systems.

2 What Is Implementation Science?

Implementation science is commonly defined as the scientific study of methods to promote the systematic uptake of evidence-based clinical treatments and practices and organisational and management interventions into routine practice.[1] It includes the study of implementation processes, intervention adaptation and fidelity, and the influences on patient, professional, and organisational behaviour. Rather than clinical effectiveness, the endpoints of interest for implementation studies are the effects of deliberate and purposive actions to implement evidence-based interventions. Acceptability, adoption, appropriateness, feasibility, fidelity, implementation cost, penetration, and sustainability are all of interest.[2] The field also encompasses research focused on the de-implementation of interventions demonstrated to be of low or no clinical benefit.[3,4] With de-implementation, a major focus is on the type of action necessary for de-implementation to occur and the time frame in which it should or can be achieved.[4]

One important question, of course, is whether implementation science is a science. Not really. The term itself is largely derived from the journal of the same name, so in reality it is a publishing construct. A search for the term 'implementation science' in PubMed reveals no use before the journal's inception in 2006. But, although it is sometimes portrayed as such, this does not make the journal's launch year zero for the field; interest in the uptake of evidence-based interventions and their sustainment in practice has a long lineage, as we describe later in this Element (see Section 3). However, having implementation science as an umbrella term has been useful, in particular in giving some coherence to what is an inherently interdisciplinary, applied research field that draws on theoretical and methodological insights across multiple well-established social science disciplines, including psychology, sociology, economics, and organisation studies. Accordingly, the study of implementation is not (or at least should not be) constrained by any particular research method.

There are of course boundaries. The focus of the field remains resolutely on the uptake of evidence-based interventions. It is, however, engaged in constant reciprocal dialogue with other fields – for example, mainstream health services research has benefited from theoretical and methodological developments in implementation science (something particularly evident in the evaluation of the effectiveness of complex interventions[5,6]). Similarly, biomedical and discovery science are increasingly interested in the role that implementation science methods could play, for example, in accelerating the translation and integration of discoveries into healthcare and ultimately health outcomes.[7]

De-implementation – efforts to remove, reduce, replace, or restrict the use of interventions that have been shown to be of no or low clinical benefit, or that are not cost-effective when compared with alternatives – is an increasing area of interest and investigation for implementation science.[3,4] Although initial theoretical work suggests that behavioural theories may not distinguish between implementation and de-implementation,[8] the factors that shape the processes of implementation and de-implementation are likely to be different and may work in different ways.[9] Frameworks for conceptualising de-implementation are now available[10,11] and, as evidence and practice experience accumulate, so will understanding of the behaviours and processes at play.

3 A Brief History of Implementation Science

Although implementation science is a contemporary term, concerns about unwarranted variation in healthcare and interest in how ideas spread in social systems have a long lineage. These issues, along with the ability to systematically codify evidence-based knowledge to enhance professional practice, have been key drivers in the development of the field.

3.1 Origins of Efforts to Understand Uptake and Reduce Unwarranted Variation

Concerns about the uptake of research findings and reducing unwarranted variation in practice and outcomes are not new. Spiegelhalter eloquently detailed the long history of enquiry into unwarranted variation in surgical outcomes initiated first in the nineteenth century by Florence Nightingale and then later championed by others, including Ernest Codman.[12] Codman advocated systematic follow-up of all patients to understand treatment outcomes, including whether errors were due to lack of 'technical knowledge or skill'.

> *To effect improvement, the first step is to admit and record the lack of perfection. The next step is to analyze the causes of failure and to determine whether these causes are controllable. We can then rationally set about effecting improvement by enforcing the control of those causes which we admit are controllable, and by directing study to methods of controlling those causes over which we now admit we have but little power.*[13]

In the 1930s, emphasis started to shift towards consideration of variation in the face of what was known to represent effective practice. Glover famously highlighted wide variation in tonsillectomy rates across England and Wales and argued that the only plausible explanation was that 'it is too often performed without adequate cause, or sufficient regard to the possibility of enlargement being temporary, physiological, or immunological'.[14]

This interest was accompanied by the development of methods to improve the quality and efficiency of healthcare, culminating in Donabedian's paradigm-shifting work on structure, process, and outcome,[15] which remains core to much of measurement in health services research. Alongside this work, Lembcke pioneered the use of audit and feedback.[16] He demonstrated that by using predetermined criteria, it was possible to collect, compare, and share data on variation in performance with clinicians in ways that could enhance the quality of care delivered. Interest in audit and feedback was rekindled in the 1980s through concerns that simply identifying suboptimal performance was in itself not sufficient to change clinicians' behaviour.[17,18] The effects of audit and feedback are among the most researched aspects of implementation science[19] (for further details, see the Element on audit, feedback, and behaviour change[20]).

3.2 Diffusion of Innovations

Alongside long-standing concerns about the need to reduce unwarranted variation, the roots of implementation science are deeply embedded within the social sciences, particularly in the literature relating to diffusion of innovations.

The history of diffusion research is well described elsewhere,[21,22] but essentially it offers a theory of how, why, and at what rate new ideas or innovations spread through defined populations and social systems. The influence of the early work of Everett Rogers in rural agriculture is well known, but it is perhaps the work of medical sociologist James Coleman that highlighted the potential of the theory, particularly to those concerned with the production and dissemination of evidence-based clinical guidelines in the late 1980s and early 1990s.

Working in the 1950s, Coleman et al.[23] investigated the adoption of the then-new antibiotic tetracycline by clinicians in Illinois. They interviewed clinicians about their use of tetracycline 15 months after the drug was introduced, and found that the social networks of participants were strongly associated with uptake.

> *... these comparisons suggest that the process of introduction for those doctors who were deeply embedded in their professional community was in fact different from the process for those who were relatively isolated from it. The highly integrated doctors seem to have learned from one another, while the less integrated ones, it seems, had each to learn afresh from the journals, the detail man (drug salesman), and other media of information.[23]*

Rogers reported that later analysis suggested more influence from advertising and pharmaceutical representatives.[21] Nevertheless, Coleman's work surfaced the potential for strategies – opinion leaders, educational outreach, and persuasive communications – that could be used to promote the uptake of research findings or, more pressingly, for codified knowledge in the form of evidence-based clinical guidelines. This became an increasing concern on both sides of the Atlantic.

3.3 Growing Interest in Getting Research Evidence into Practice

The early period of evidence-based medicine focused on producing and synthesising research evidence, on making it more accessible, and on promoting its use in the development of clinical guidelines. This required the creation of methods and supporting evidence infrastructures. In the late 1980s, the RAND Corporation were pioneers of systematic and standardised processes to assess health technologies.[24] Also in the USA, the Agency for Health Care Policy and Research was established in 1989 to enhance the quality, appropriateness, and effectiveness of healthcare services.[25] These early iterations of what has become known as health technology assessment is now a mainstay of health systems globally and one of the key building blocks of evidence-based clinical guidelines.

Alongside the systematic codification of knowledge, there was renewed and increasing interest in getting the presented evidence to be adopted and used in practice. In Canada, Lomas et al. were recognising that guidelines alone were unlikely to effect change in actual practice.[26,27] In the USA, Soumerai et al. were investigating strategies to improve the prescribing practices of primary care clinicians.[28] And in Europe, Grol[29] and Grimshaw and Russell[30] were exploring how best to implement clinical guidelines in primary care.

In 1994, the Agency for Health Care Policy and Research convened a conference of experts, including Everett Rogers, to discuss and provide guidance on effective methods of guideline dissemination.[31] At the same time, in the UK these ideas were also being shared with mass audiences in the National Health Service (NHS) via the groundbreaking *Effective Health Care* series of bulletins – first through *Implementing clinical practice guidelines*[32] in 1994 and then later through *Getting evidence into practice*.[33] The *Effective Health Care* bulletins, which were produced by the University of York and began in 1992, predated the creation in 1999 of a national guideline infrastructure in the form of the National Institute for Clinical Excellence (NICE). The bulletins were charged with synthesising and disseminating the best available evidence on selected topics to inform NHS policy and practice.

The 1999 *Getting evidence into practice* bulletin was one of the first publications to advocate, albeit somewhat naïvely, for theoretically informed implementation.[33] More rigorous and systematic approaches to theory development and application were to follow, most notably led by Michie and Johnston.[34] Underpinning these approaches was the principle that because evidence-based practice depends on human behaviour, change efforts could be improved by drawing on theories of behaviour change.[34] Advocacy for and use of theoretical approaches to understand, guide, and evaluate implementation processes was one of the key pre-existing principles from which a new general field of implementation science would emerge. With the launch of the journal *Implementation Science* in 2006,[1] the field finally had a focal point for its outputs.

3.4 Evolution and Investment in Implementation Studies As a Research Field

Globally, significant investment in research funding and training now supports the field of implementation. The past decade has seen an increase in dedicated, standalone training courses and, most recently, more formal doctoral-level courses. These often adapt and apply methods that are drawn from spheres such as clinical epidemiology, health services research, sociology, and psychology to implementation science questions.[35,36] This growth in bespoke training has led in turn to the emergence of researchers who now define themselves as implementation scientists rather than as working within a particular discipline.

The other significant investment has been in research infrastructure. As the potential of implementation science methods has become increasingly recognised, the need to harness the expertise and resources of the field in continuous efforts to improve healthcare systems has also been acknowledged. This recognition has led to the development of new models of research and practice partnerships. In the USA, the Veterans Health Administration has long been at the forefront of efforts to enhance partnered research through its Health Services Research and Development Service and the Quality Enhancement Research Initiative (QUERI).[37] Since 1998, QUERI collaborations have identified service gaps and developed evidence-based best practices, embedding them into routine practice across the Veterans Health Administration system.[38] The key feature of QUERI has been a strong focus on rigorous comparative effectiveness research and the evaluation of implementation strategies to support uptake and spread. This approach has been mirrored in other geographical settings, most notably in the UK through Collaborations for Leadership in Applied Health Research and Care (CLAHRCs), which were launched in 2008 and funded by the National Institute for Health Research.

CLAHRCs were collaborative partnerships between universities and surrounding health service organisations and were focused on improving patient outcomes through the conduct and application of applied health research. Although CLAHRCs generated a large body of knowledge and learning, the relative lack of national impact on healthcare provision or outcomes has been noted.[39] The policy shift from CLARHCs to Applied Research Collaborations (ARCs) in 2019 suggests efforts to address this. With a clearer focus on high-quality applied health and care research, ARCs may be closer to the QUERI initiative in both form and function.

4 Implementation Science in Action

Traditionally, implementation science has three areas of focus. First, it encompasses theory and research focused on exploring the contexts, behaviours, and practices that can act as influences on successful implementation, specifically exploring barriers and enablers. Second, there is a focus on the design and evaluation of strategies to address those factors identified as helping or hindering the implementation of evidence-based interventions in a given context. Finally, the field features an increasing focus on understanding the process of implementation itself: what actually gets implemented and how, the intended and unintended mechanisms of strategies (how and why they work or do not work), the influence of context on implementation efforts, and ultimately the sustainability of interventions that are implemented.

In all implementation efforts, there is a need for someone somewhere to do something differently.[40] In order to achieve this, a clear understanding is required of what needs to change and the factors that are likely to help or hinder any change to occur. These influencing factors could be related to:

- the nature of the intervention, practice, or policy to be introduced
- the place where change will occur
- the people involved
- the processes and resources required to ensure that change occurs
- the influence of the wider economic, political, and social environment.

Identifying and understanding the likely influencing factors is now a core function of developmental studies in implementation research, and a large evidence base now exists. Helpfully, insights on clearly defined barriers and enablers have been synthesised in a range of sectors. For example, digital health is an area of increasing implementation focus, but it is also an area where there is considerable convergence across studies on the key factors that influence implementation.[41] Ross et al.'s review of systematic reviews highlights the need for adequate infrastructure, engagement of key personnel, organisational readiness, and the fit of digital innovations with workflows, processes, and systems.[41] These insights are essential to inform the design of appropriate implementation strategies.

4.1 Implementation Strategies

Implementation strategies are designed and deployed to bring about changes in healthcare organisations, the behaviour of healthcare professionals, or the use of health services by healthcare recipients.[42] Put simply, they represent the 'how to' element of any change initiative.[43] A large number of implementation strategies have been documented, notably by the Cochrane Effective Practice and Organisation of Care group, and they have long been deemed to be an essential driver for bringing about change in healthcare practice.[27,43]

The literature has explored the effectiveness of a wide range of strategies, including those targeting the behaviour of individual professionals, those targeting an organisation, and/or those targeting the wider policy context. Table 1 presents a summary of strategies commonly used in healthcare practice, the features that enable their successful implementation, and findings

Table 1 Commonly used implementation strategies, their enabling features, and evidence of effects

Strategy	Enabling features	Evidence of effects
Audit and feedback[19,44]	In areas where baseline performance is low, feedback is provided by a supervisor or colleague more than once, is delivered in both verbal and written formats, and includes explicit performance targets and an action plan.	Consistent small to moderate effects when optimally designed.
Computerised reminders[45,46]	Automated on-screen reminders to prescribe specific medications, to warn about drug interactions, to provide vaccinations, or to order tests.	Consistent small to moderate effects for simple one-step prescribing and decisions about which tests to order.
Educational meetings[47]	Meetings utilising mixed (interactive and didactic) formats, and focusing on issues/outcomes likely to be perceived as priorities. Meetings did not appear to be effective for complex behaviours and were less effective for less serious outcomes.	Small to moderate effects BUT poor reporting of interventions limits understanding of optimal configurations.
Educational outreach[48]	Visits by credible and trained people to professionals in their own setting to provide information on performance and how to change. Face-to-face visits that occur as part of a sustained effort to improve practices appear to be more effective than one-time efforts.	Consistent small to moderate effects for improving prescribing practices and test ordering.

Facilitation[49,50]	Combination of external experts and internal facilitators applying a range of enabling skills and improvement strategies to implement change in a practice setting. Project management skills and ability to engage and manage relationships between key agents and to identify and negotiate barriers to implementation found to be key. Often resource intensive.	Small to moderate effects BUT evidence lacking on optimal characteristics of facilitation.
Financial incentives[51,52]	Financial incentives and pay-for-performance schemes that target professional, group, or organisational-level behaviours may improve processes of care, but benefits on patient outcomes are less clear. Impact on processes of care is most likely in those that are relatively simple to measure, have room for improvement, and are deemed to be achievable.	Small effects on processes of care reported BUT design limitations of studies limit certainty.
Local opinion leaders[53]	In combination with other strategies, opinion leaders can enhance the tendency of healthcare professionals to follow evidence-based guidelines. Potential resource implications relating to identification, training, and sustainability.	Consistent small to moderate effects BUT poor reporting limits understanding of how and why strategy is effective.

Table 1 (cont.)

Strategy	Enabling features	Evidence of effects
Printed educational materials[54]	Delivered personally, through mass mailings, or passively delivered through broader communication channels (e.g. available on the internet). Can improve practice when there is a single clear message, if the change is relatively simple to accomplish, and there is consensus that a change in practice is required. Can be widely distributed at relatively low costs.	Small effects when optimally designed and targeted.
Quality improvement collaboratives[55,56]	Core enablers include having teams from multiple healthcare organisations come together to iteratively learn, apply, and share improvement methods, best practices, and performance data on a clearly defined improvement goal. Often resource intensive.	Small to substantial effects reported BUT design and reporting limitations of studies and likely publication bias limit certainty.

on their effects.[19,44–56] A more comprehensive classification of implementation strategies has been compiled by the Expert Recommendations for Implementing Change project.[57] At first sight, many of the strategies presented in Table 1 look similar to each other, but there are nuanced differences in the approaches taken. For example, one can argue that facilitation is about helping people to change, while opinion leaders influence people to change, and educational outreach can be described as a form of peer-led review of performance.

With small to moderate effects reported across strategies, no single approach appears to be more effective across settings and contexts. Although evidence has accumulated over the past 30 years and synthesis methods have improved, there is much similarity between the summary of findings presented in Table 1 and those of the early reviews of implementation strategies. Those early reviews indicated that while there were no magic bullets for improving the quality of healthcare, a range of interventions were available that, if used appropriately, could lead to improvements in professional practice.[58,59]

This led to suggestions that, despite a growing literature, the science around strategies had stagnated,[60] and such concerns have since seen efforts shift away from rudimentary replication studies to a research agenda that focuses on understanding the underlying mechanisms of action[61] in order to better tailor and optimise interventions to maximise their effects.[62–64]

Although implementation strategies are often presented as discrete or single entities, this is not always the most accurate description. For example, Box 1 shows that an educational outreach strategy, which was deployed to reduce prescribing errors in general practices in England, was actually part of an intervention that was both complex and multifaceted.[65] In their seminal review of guideline dissemination and implementation strategies, Grimshaw et al. found that nearly three-quarters of included studies were in fact evaluations of interventions deploying multiple strategies.[66]

Many early trials of implementation strategies could be considered to have been designed using Martin Eccles's famous ISLAGIATT maxim: 'It seemed like a good idea at the time.' Some strategies suffered from being poorly conceived: little thought was given in the initial stages to the behaviours or processes that needed to be targeted for change to occur, or to whether or not the strategy deployed would (or could) address any underlying factors. Strategies have also often been inconsistently labelled, poorly described, and lacking in sufficient detail to guide their use. This has led to calls for more detailed specification of both the strategies themselves and the behaviours to be targeted in order to ensure greater alignment between intervention components and measured outcomes.[40,43] Box 2 provides an overview of two useful frameworks, one for informing strategy selection and intervention

Box 1 Using educational outreach to reduce medication errors in primary care

The PINCER trial – a pharmacist-led intervention comprising electronic feedback, educational outreach, and dedicated support – was found to be more effective than simple computerised reminders for reducing a range of medication errors in general practice.[65] The PINCER intervention was multifaceted, and activities included:

- using software to search clinical systems to identify patients at risk of hazardous prescribing
- conducting reviews of patient records and prescribed medication
- the pharmacist meeting members of the practice team to discuss the computer-generated feedback on patients with medication errors
- ongoing dedicated pharmacist support, using the principles of educational outreach and root cause analysis, to provide education and feedback on medication errors in practice
- working with practices to appoint an internal lead, and then establish and implement a practice action plan to resolve issues identified and prevent recurrence
- inviting patients into the surgery for a medication review with the pharmacist, or a member of the general practice team, with the aim of correcting errors.

design, and one for specifying the behaviour change needed. Both have utility for implementation in practice and provide much-needed guidance on strategy selection.

Attention has also focused on gaining greater understanding of the influence of context where an evidence-based intervention is introduced. A narrow focus on what works, in isolation from the wider economic, political, and social environment within which implementation will occur, is recognised as no longer being sufficient for causal explanation. Rather, implementation is better understood as a critical event in a system that can lead to new understandings, displacement of existing practices, and the evolution of new processes.[67] This understanding acknowledges that the context in which implementation takes place is not static but dynamic. Health systems are not fixed organisational structures or entities; rather, they are unfolding and evolutionary, and go through continuous adaptions, so they require constant work to be held together.[68] As the two frameworks in Box 2 highlight, an

BOX 2 TWO TOOLS TO INFORM STRATEGY SELECTION AND INTENDED BEHAVIOUR CHANGE

Proctor et al.'s Framework for Specifying Behaviour[43]

- **Name it:** name the strategy, preferably using language that is consistent with existing literature.
- **Define it:** define the implementation strategy and any discrete components operationally.
- **Specify it:**

  ◦ identify who enacts the strategy (e.g. managers, professionals, patients, etc.)
  ◦ specify the precise actions, steps, or processes that need to be enacted
  ◦ specify the intended targets of the strategy (i.e. what are we trying to change?)
  ◦ specify when the strategy is used
  ◦ specify the dosage of the implementation strategy
  ◦ identify and measure the implementation outcome(s) likely to be affected
  ◦ provide empirical, theoretical, or pragmatic justification for the choice of strategy.

Action, Actor, Context, Target, Time (AACTT) Framework for Specifying Behaviour Change[40]

- **Action:** specify the behaviour that needs to change, in terms that can be observed or measured.
- **Actor:** specify the person/people that do(es) or could do the action targeted.
- **Context:** specify the physical location, emotional context, or social setting in which the action is performed.
- **Target:** specify the person/people with/for whom the action is performed.
- **Time:** specify when the action is performed (the time/date/frequency).

understanding of the context of implementation is an essential prerequisite for strategy selection.

Given all this, there is a case for arguing that the general principles for strategy selection first outlined by Grol nearly 30 years ago – that it should be planned on several levels and that strategies should be directed to the specific barriers to change for specific target groups – still hold true.[29]

4.2 Theories and Frameworks in Implementation Science

Choice of implementation strategy is likely to be best informed by the nature of the change desired and an informed assessment of how and why a specific strategy is expected to be effective in a given context. Theory provides an essential lens through which we can anticipate, identify, and describe the key features that will influence change. The use of theory helps to clarify the nature of the change required, together with consideration of the wider system, process, and contextual features that need to be addressed if plans for implementation are to be successful. There is now no shortage of implementation frameworks and theories.[69,70] (Indeed, one of the less helpful developments in the field over the past decade has been a proliferation of 'me too' process models and determinant frameworks, many of which are similarly theoretically grounded, share common antecedents, and apply similar constructs.)

These theories and frameworks can be used to guide the process of translating research into practice, to understand or explain what influences implementation outcomes, or to evaluate implementation efforts generally. Table 2 describes six commonly used theories and frameworks in implementation science. All six have broad utility and can be thought of as evaluation frameworks because they all specify concepts and constructs that may be put into operation and measured. Though a plethora of options exist, this represents a core list through which nearly all implementation issues and questions can be addressed and assessed.

Theory or framework selection can be challenging. As theories and frameworks vary in purpose, complexity, and intended targets, practitioners have reported struggling to identify and select appropriate frameworks to guide implementation in practice.[83] In response to this, practical guides are now available to facilitate the use of frameworks beyond the research setting.[84–87] Box 3 highlights a pragmatic approach to theory selection proposed by Lynch et al.,[85] which seeks to encourage the use of theory to guide implementation in practice.

4.3 Implementation Science in Practice

As this section has illustrated, a large and growing body of evidence on implementation now exists. But, as a research-based discipline, many important messages remain buried in the literature and have yet to disseminate out to routine practice. The shift from CLAHRCs to ARCs (see Section 3.4) is a reflection of growing recognition of the need to better harness the expertise and resources of the field in efforts to improve healthcare.

Models of research and practice partnerships, such as ARCs, are increasingly viewed as integral to the development of learning health systems,[38] which seek

Table 2 Commonly used implementation theories and frameworks

Theory or framework	Defining characteristics	Application
Consolidated Framework for Implementation Research (CFIR)[71,72]	Grounded in diffusion of innovations theory,[21] the five domains in CFIR represent 38 constructs relating to the planned intervention, the immediate and wider contexts where the implementation activities will occur, the individuals involved, and the process of delivering the actual intervention.	Understanding and explaining what influences implementation outcomes and evaluating implementation efforts.
COM-B[73]	Implementation of evidence-based practice and public health depends on behaviour change, and behaviour is the result of an interaction between three components: **c**apability, **o**pportunity, and **m**otivation. Capability and opportunity can influence motivation, while enacting a behaviour can alter capability, opportunity, and motivation.	Understanding and explaining what influences implementation outcomes and evaluating implementation efforts.
Promoting Action on Research Implementation in Health Services (PARIHS)[49,74,75]	Successful implementation is a function of the interaction of three core elements – the strength and nature of the evidence, the context or environment into which the evidence is used, and how implementation is facilitated. The PARIHS framework was later revised so that facilitation was recognised as the active ingredient assessing, aligning, and integrating the other three constructs (innovation, recipients, and context).	Understanding and explaining what influences implementation outcomes and evaluating implementation efforts.

Table 2 (cont.)

Theory or framework	Defining characteristics	Application
Normalisation Process Theory (NPT)[76,77]	NPT facilitates understanding of the extent to which new processes become part of routine practice. NPT comprises four main constructs, representing individual and collective levels of work involved in the implementation of new practice: coherence, cognitive participation, collective action, and reflexive monitoring.	Understanding and explaining what influences implementation outcomes and evaluating implementation efforts.
RE-AIM[78,79]	Originally developed as a framework for consistent reporting of public health and health promotion research. RE-AIM is a planning and evaluation framework of five constructs deemed important to impact and sustainability: **r**each, **e**ffectiveness, **a**doption, **i**mplementation, and **m**aintenance.	Guiding the process of implementation and evaluating implementation outcomes.
Theoretical Domains Framework (TDF)[80,81]	TDF is an integrated theoretical framework synthesised from 128 theoretical constructs (from 33 theories) which were judged most relevant to implementation.[82] TDF is organised into 14 theoretical domains of constructs that influence behaviour. Often used in conjunction with COM-B.	Understanding and explaining what influences implementation outcomes. Most often used in intervention development.

Box 3 QUESTIONS TO HELP SELECT A THEORY OR FRAMEWORK TO GUIDE THE PLANNING,
DOING, AND EVALUATION OF IMPLEMENTATION

- **Who are you working with: individuals, teams, or wider settings?**
  Consider the fit of the theoretical approaches to the organisational level where your project is positioned, and whether more than one approach is required to guide implementation at different levels.

- **When in the process are you going to use the theory?**
  Some approaches lend themselves particularly to design and planning, others to the process of implementation, and others to evaluating implementation success.

- **Why are you applying a theory?**
  What is your aim, and what do you need to understand? Does the theory need to help with gaining a better understanding of barriers and enablers, to develop knowledge about an ongoing implementation process, or to provide a framework of relevant implementation outcomes?

- **How will you collect data?**
  Choice of theoretical approach may be informed by what data will be available for analysis.

- **What resources are available?**
  The number of staff and the time available to them to participate in the implementation project should be considered.

Adapted from Lynch et al.[85]

to improve care through a continuous cycle of knowledge production and implementation (see the Element on learning health systems[88]). The trailblazer for such initiatives is the QUERI initiative of the US Veterans Health Administration, mentioned in Section 3.4.[38] A system-wide approach to accelerating the adoption of research-based knowledge, QUERI has long recognised that although there are key differences between doing implementation (i.e. actually putting into practice new evidence-based policies, procedures, or approaches) and undertaking research on implementation, both require infrastructure to ensure capacity and capability.

Box 4 highlights the step-based QUERI framework used to systematically identify and develop evidence-based practices and to embed these into routine practice across the Veterans Health Administration system.[37] As can be seen,

---

Box 4 IMPLEMENTATION SCIENCE IN ACTION – THE QUERI PROCESS

(1) Identify high-risk/high-volume/high-burden diseases or problems for veterans.

(2) Identify evidence-based guidelines, recommendations, and best practices.

(3) Explore existing practice patterns and outcomes across the Veterans Health Administration and any current variation from identified best practices.

(4) Identify and implement interventions to promote best practices.

- Undertake systematic searches for implementation interventions, change strategies, and related tools.
- Develop/adapt and evaluate implementation of strategies or practice support tools.

(5) Document that best practices improve outcomes.

(6) Document that outcomes are associated with improved health-related quality of life.

Adapted from Stetler et al.[37] More detail on resources and tools can be found on the QUERI website;[89] *Implementation Science* has also published a QUERI theme series of articles.[90]

---

this offers an explicit series of steps for first identifying and then addressing practice variations within a health system, as well as simultaneously generating new knowledge and learning. A key feature of QUERI is its strong focus on rigorous comparative effectiveness research, particularly through the evaluation of implementation strategies to support uptake and spread. Since its inception, hundreds of studies have been conducted to inform the organisation and delivery of a wide range of evidence-based services, including mental health, substance abuse services, and diabetes prevention.[38,91]

QUERI can be viewed largely as a research-based initiative, but its strength is that it is fully embedded in a health system and harnesses the principles of co-production in the creation and implementation of research-based knowledge. Implementation efforts are therefore truly a research-practice partnership. As QUERI has developed, focus has increased on the development of research tools and methods to support implementation efforts in practice, and on building system capacity and capability to support primary data collection and foster organisational readiness for change. Infrastructure on this scale not only needs adequate year-on-year funding but also requires a significant commitment to investment in the longer term. It is not surprising, therefore, that the most recent developments in the QUERI framework have focused on ensuring that the impacts of implementation efforts are captured in ways that can facilitate operational understanding of the value of investment on this scale.[92]

5 Critiques of Implementation Science

Implementation science continues to mature, which is manifest in the growing number of contributions offering critical reflections on the current state of the field. This section will provide a brief overview of the main themes emerging from these critiques. We will start by reflecting on the extent to which implementation science can be considered a truly multidisciplinary and interdisciplinary field (Section 5.1). This will be followed by a discussion of the tensions involved in studying complex interventions in diverse implementation contexts (Section 5.2). We will conclude by outlining criticisms of implementation science as an applied discipline which, although it has an explicit mission to improve patient care, has not always been successful in bridging the gap between research and practice (Section 5.3).

5.1 Implementation Science as a Multidisciplinary and Interdisciplinary Field

Implementation science is an inherently multidisciplinary and interdisciplinary field. It draws, as we have mentioned, on theoretical and methodological insights from many disciplines and offers tools for studying implementation at different levels of analysis. However, interdisciplinary thinking is not always apparent in empirical implementation studies. Overall, cross-fertilisation with other social science disciplines remains relatively limited and somewhat unequal. Ideas imported from other fields still tend to be dominated by approaches derived from evidence-based medicine and behavioural psychology, which have been particularly influential in implementation science.[93]

Broadly interdisciplinary origins of implementation science, on the one hand, and the predominance of certain disciplinary and epistemological ways of thinking, on the other, make an uneasy combination. This results in a number of tensions. Approaches focusing on group, organisational, and systemic levels of analysis tend to be less utilised than individual educational and psychological approaches. Implementation researchers and practitioners may stubbornly adhere to their preferred methodological orientations, regardless of the nature of the implementation issue or contextual barriers to be addressed. At the same time, the development of some implementation scientists as disciplinary agnostics may cause other difficulties because they may lack in-depth training in core social science disciplines and have a relatively limited methodological and theoretical repertoire on which to draw. As a result, identified implementation problems may not match with the chosen change approaches to address them, and implementation strategies may be poorly tailored to their contexts.[64,94]

Implementation science could benefit from a broader dialogue with a variety of philosophical and theoretical orientations. This would enable diversification of its epistemological assumptions, conceptual lenses, and methodological approaches.[95] Table 3 provides examples of diverse approaches that could be helpful for addressing implementation questions that have so far been overshadowed by the field's predominantly positivist agenda. Some of these intellectual traditions, such as critical realism and complexity theory, have already entered the discipline. The adoption of other, less familiar approaches has the potential to lead to the development of novel perspectives on implementation. Engagement with these strands of thinking must, however, take into account their underlying philosophical and disciplinary roots as well as the internal logic and assumptions. Multidisciplinary training programmes for implementation scientists should therefore consider offering in-depth training in at least one core social science discipline, which may require a fine balancing act between multidisciplinary versatility and professional specialisation.

5.2 Implementation Science as a Study of Complex Interventions in Diverse Contexts

One of the recent trends is the increasing complexity and variability of implementation interventions that unfold in diverse and changing contexts. As we described in Section 4, these interventions often comprise multiple, interrelated components and may target several levels within a health system. The traditional focus on what works (i.e. did intervention X lead to outcome Y?) is no longer sufficient for causal explanation (i.e. how, why, and under what circumstances did intervention X lead to outcome Y?).[63] Although process evaluations of implementation interventions are now becoming increasingly routine,[77] implementation science has, to date, often offered relatively little understanding as to *how* different implementation strategies work – that is, the specific mechanisms through which they influence delivery

Table 3 Intellectual traditions and relevance of their central questions to implementation science

Perspective	Disciplinary roots	Questions relevant to implementation science	Potential implications for the practice of implementation
Ethnography	Anthropology	What is the culture of a certain group of people (e.g. an organisation) involved in implementation? How does it manifest in the process of implementation?	Observing the behaviour of people in organisations or communities involved in implementation in order to reveal hidden barriers.
Critical realism	Philosophy, social sciences, and evaluation	What are the causal mechanisms explaining how and why implementation unfolds as it does in a particular context?	Eliciting, comparing, and refining stakeholders' theories of change or programme theories behind each implementation intervention.
Constructivism	Sociology	What are the implementation actors' reported perceptions, explanations, beliefs, and world views? What consequences do these have on implementation?	Comparing the perceptions of multiple implementation stakeholders with one another and with those of funders or commissioners; interpreting the effects of differences in perceptions on attainment of intervention goals.
Phenomenology	Philosophy	What is the meaning, structure, and essence of the lived experience of implementation for a certain group of people?	Understanding how patients, families, and carers make sense of participation in implementation interventions.

Table 3 (cont.)

Perspective	Disciplinary roots	Questions relevant to implementation science	Potential implications for the practice of implementation
Symbolic interactionism	Social psychology	What common set of symbols and understandings has emerged to give meaning to people's interactions in the process of implementation?	Understanding what is most important to people from organisations and communities involved in an intervention, what will need to change for successful implementation, and what will generate most resistance.
Semiotics	Linguistics	How do signs (i.e. words and symbols) carry and convey meaning in different implementation contexts?	Using texts and images persuasively to communicate key messages, overcome resistance, and assist implementation.
Narrative analysis	Social sciences, literary criticism	What do stories of implementation reveal about implementation actors and contexts?	Learning from stories of successful and unsuccessful implementation, as told by different stakeholders.
Complexity theory	Theoretical physics, natural sciences	How can the emergent and non-linear dynamics of implementation and its context be captured and understood?	Quick and effective adaptation of an ongoing implementation intervention in response to its dynamic context.

| Critical theory | Political philosophy | How do the experiences of inequality, injustice, and subjugation shape implementation? | Challenging the traditional dominance of researchers and senior organisational stakeholders by giving voices to those with less power, such as service users and junior staff. |
| Feminist inquiry | Interdisciplinary | How does the lens of gender shape and affect our understanding and actions in the process of implementation? | Addressing the issues of inequality and injustice affecting women in the process of implementation; developing inclusive, collaborative, and participatory implementation approaches. |

Adapted from Kislov et al.[95] and Patton.[96]

of care.[64,97] One possible explanation is that knowledge about processes derived from past interventions is not applied to the development or evaluation of new ones. There is also, speaking more broadly, a problem of one trend replacing another without carrying forward the previous lessons learnt.[64,94,97]

Another explanation for the current lack of understanding of how different interventions work relates to the dominant patterns of conceptual work in the discipline. Implementation science has been criticised for favouring determinant frameworks and process models. Determinant frameworks, such as the Consolidated Framework for Implementation Research[71] and the Theoretical Domains Framework,[80] describe types, classes, or domains of factors that act as either barriers or enablers to successful implementation. Process models, such as the knowledge-to-action cycle,[98] neatly divide an idealised implementation process into a series of phases or stages. Such models and frameworks can helpfully alert researchers to the range of components that should be accounted for in intervention design and evaluation. At the same time, they have a tendency to oversimplify, reducing complex relationships between interventions, implementers, and contexts to prescriptive checklists or stages. Relatively little attention is paid to explicating functional relationships between different determinants, causal mechanisms through which different stages of implementation or contextual variables influence outcomes, or additional mediators and moderators affecting these causal pathways.[64]

These issues matter for a number of reasons. First, identification of enablers and barriers is only the first step in an implementation journey and is not sufficient for making informed decisions about which implementation strategies should be deployed to address different configurations of determinants. Second, successful implementation is contingent on collective action of multiple implementation actors, such as researchers, managers, and clinicians, who constantly adjust the process of implementation in response to an ever-changing context rather than follow a pre-planned sequence of actions. Finally, some of the best explanations are 'mechanism-based',[95] detailing the cogs and wheels of the causal processes through which implementation outcomes are brought about.[67,97,99]

Box 5 shows how mechanism-based thinking has been applied by different teams to the study of facilitation – an implementation strategy that relies on a designated role (facilitator) encouraging others to reflect upon their current practices to identify gaps in performance, introduce change, enable knowledge sharing, and thus improve outcomes.[101] This example highlights the benefits of focusing on relationships and interdependencies between a relatively limited

Box 5 Applying a mechanism-based approach to the study of facilitation

Mechanism-Based Explanation in Conceptual Work on Facilitation

Berta et al.[100] suggest that facilitation acts through stimulating higher-order learning (i.e. analysis, evaluation, and reflection) through experimenting with, generating knowledge about, and sustaining small-scale adaptations to organisational processes.

Mechanism-Based Explanation in Qualitative Longitudinal Research on Facilitation

Kislov et al.[101] describe three mechanisms that may lead to *distortion* of facilitation over time, if it is adapted in an uncritical and uncontrolled way. These mechanisms are:

- prioritisation of (measurable) outcomes over the (interactive) process
- reduction of (multi-professional) team engagement
- erosion of the facilitator role: shift from *facilitating* to *doing* implementation.

Mechanism-Based Explanation in the Context of a Randomised Controlled Trial (RCT)

A pragmatic clustered RCT of facilitation used to implement evidence-based urinary incontinence recommendations in nursing care showed no statistically significant differences in primary outcome (compliance with continence recommendation between standard dissemination and two different approaches to facilitation).[102] An embedded process evaluation[103] identified four mechanisms underpinning the success of facilitation in those sites where it worked well:

- alignment of the intervention with the needs and expectations of facilitators and their organisations
- prioritisation of organisational involvement in both the study and the facilitation programme
- collective engagement with the facilitation intervention by managers, facilitators, and other staff
- sustained learning over time.

number of elements, such as organisational factors, characteristics of facilitators, and collective processes underpinning facilitation. Mechanism-based explanations presented here shed light on how the interplay between participating entities (i.e. individuals, teams, and organisations), their properties (i.e. roles, expectations, and experiences), and activities (i.e. alignment, prioritisation, engagement, and learning) produces the effect of interest (i.e. successful or unsuccessful facilitation).[99]

This example suggests that intervention fidelity should be defined *functionally* in relation to fit with the underlying causal mechanisms (i.e. what processes does the intervention initiate and how?), rather than *compositionally* (i.e. what is the composition, dose, and frequency of the intervention?).[104] It also shows that flexible longitudinal designs can be invaluable for exploring causal pathways and uncovering the emergent and dynamic aspects of implementation.

Adopting a mechanism-based approach can also lead to a more nuanced understanding and capturing of implementation outcomes, which otherwise might remain rather crude,[94] as well as to a better integration of formative and summative evaluation findings.[6,94] Lewis et al. argue that more attention should be paid to proximal implementation outcomes that occur as a direct result of a specific mechanism of action.[97] For instance, the strategy of facilitation acts through the mechanism of *enabling group learning* on the proximal outcomes of *knowledge* and *skills* to influence distal outcomes of *clinical behaviour* or *patient satisfaction*. Identification of proximal outcomes can be guided by asking: 'How will I know if this implementation strategy had an effect via the mechanism that I think it is activating?'

By contrast, distal intervention outcomes – that is, those that an implementation process is ultimately intended to achieve – are not the most immediate elements in the causal pathway.[97] Examples include changes in frequency of certain clinical behaviours or improvements in patients' symptoms. While such indicators are often extremely informative, they do not necessarily reflect the actual use of research knowledge in healthcare practice for a number of reasons.

- The steps between implementation interventions and distal outcomes may be numerous, making interpretation of causality difficult, especially when causal pathways that make complex interventions work remain unclear.[94]
- Taking research knowledge into account when making decisions does not always mean that this knowledge will be *implemented* in practice.[94] For instance, research evidence can – justifiably – be overridden by individual patient preferences.

- Engagement with new knowledge may lead to subtle and gradual changes in identities, emotions, and discourses that are difficult to measure but can still shape individual behaviours and collective practices.[105]

One promising avenue for future methodological research could involve design and validation of a new generation of measures that would capture uptake of valuable knowledge, skills, and practices. This may include a range of intermediate indicators closely linked to the mechanisms through which interventions work.[2] When designing new measures, it is also important to remember that implementation strategies are not without costs and compete with other healthcare activities for finite resources.[106] More economic evaluation would advance the ability to understand which strategies might be suitable for different contexts and whether improvements in implementation are worth the added costs (see the Element on health economics[107]). This remains a neglected area of inquiry for the field as whole.[108,109]

5.3 Implementation Science as an Applied Field

Implementation science is an inherently applied field of inquiry. Its knowledge base has been accumulated with an explicit aim of guiding knowledge translation and achieving positive impact on the outcomes of implementation strategies. A significant and increasing body of published research on how to support implementation now exists. However, much of this learning remains 'locked up' within the academic community, perversely perpetuating the very same research and practice gap that implementation science has pledged to address. This is not particularly surprising as implementation scientists often operate within institutional structures, which tend to prioritise high-quality academic outputs over generation of pragmatic insights or evidence-based lessons learnt.

Implementation research outputs are mostly written for fellow academics and reflect their preoccupations with methodological rigour, originality, and novelty. Clinicians, managers, and policy-makers (subsequently referred to as 'practitioners') are likely to find the following aspects of this development particularly frustrating.

- There has been a massive proliferation of theories, models, and frameworks on implementation and knowledge translation. But many have not been applied and tested in more than one study.[94]
- Pressures to generate novel contributions may promote 'pseudoinnovation':[110] new implementation models and frameworks often ignore previously published

work, reinventing concepts and repackaging what is already known under new labels.[94,110]

- Insufficient detail in reporting implementation interventions (e.g. why they were selected, how they were tailored to contextual determinants, what causal pathways they were supposed to activate to achieve outcomes, and how their components were enacted in practice) complicates their practical assessment, replication, and application in new settings.[61,64]

Evaluations of effectiveness (what works) and determinants of change (what elements of context facilitate or hinder implementation), both of which are evident in the mainstream literature, are not necessarily sufficient for addressing practical concerns. What practitioners also want to know is how to address their practical problems by selecting and designing an implementation intervention, how to make this intervention work in practice in the face of numerous obstacles, and how to rapidly evaluate its success. The publication of pragmatic guides helping practitioners to choose between different theories, models, and frameworks to inform their implementation projects is a valuable development in this regard.[85,87] Elicitation of stakeholders' programme theories and explication of mechanisms can, in principle, also generate shared understandings and practically applicable knowledge.[111] However, if these remain exclusively driven by the agenda of researchers, benefits for practitioners will not necessarily materialise.

At a more fundamental level, many of these issues can be addressed by collaborative research partnerships,[39] implementation laboratories,[112] and other co-production arrangements that bring together researchers and non-researchers. Much practical, experiential knowledge is collectively generated as part of these increasingly popular collaborative approaches.[113] However, uptake of co-production in implementation science is not without problems.

First, co-produced, practice-oriented knowledge is rarely captured in codified form and thus may fail to be transferred and applied beyond its original setting. The existing body of work, which tends to target researchers, may therefore need to be complemented by publicly accessible literature with a more pragmatic how-to-do focus. This will require a significant input from practitioners.

Second, despite the rhetoric of improving patient care, the co-design and co-production of implementation studies with patients remains relatively rare, with more attention being paid to collaboration with clinicians and managers within healthcare organisations.[39] Patients, carers, and families impact on the variability and outcomes of interventions, in effect often becoming co-creators of implementation, and can provide unique insights in supporting design and evaluation.[114]

Finally, despite significant investment in co-produced forms of working on implementation, many methods for stakeholder involvement are poorly specified, their advantages are often taken for granted, and critical evaluation of their application in practice is missing. Wensing and Grol argue, for instance, that 'it is unclear how available research evidence and theory is combined with stakeholder involvement, if stakeholders have suggestions that contradict existing knowledge'.[94] More critical and programmatic research into the processes, practices, and impacts of co-produced implementation strategies is therefore a promising area for future development of implementation science as a field. (This is explored further in the Element on co-producing and co-designing.[115])

In summary, multiple barriers to knowledge flows exist between different intellectual traditions, between approaches focusing on determinants, mechanisms, and outcomes of implementation, and between the interests of researchers, practitioners, and service users. Table 4 outlines steps that can be taken to facilitate learning across these boundaries and thus realise the potential of implementation science to contribute to solving real-world healthcare problems in the interest of patients and populations. However, only through joint working that brings together all implementation stakeholders can this learning lead to translating the science of implementation into practice.

6 Conclusions

The past 20 years has witnessed growing global interest in methods to enhance the uptake of research findings into healthcare practice and policy. This interest has fuelled the funding of infrastructure and an ever-growing community of dedicated researchers. Implementation science has much to offer improvement efforts in routine practice. The field offers rigorous evaluation methods and theoretical approaches that can be harnessed to design, facilitate, and understand the uptake of evidence-based interventions into practice.

A large and burgeoning body of evidence on adoption, diffusion, and implementation (and increasingly de-implementation) now exists, but challenges remain. Many important messages remain buried within the literature and their use in and influence on routine healthcare practice could be greater. Implementation science as a field is at the end of the beginning. The immediate challenge for the field is not just to get research findings into practice but also to get implementation science into practice.

Table 4 Directions for future development of implementation science as an applied field

Desired practice	Possible strategies
Cross-fertilisation between different disciplines, theoretical orientations, and implementation methodologies	• Broadening the range of questions addressed by implementation science to better reflect the needs of health services and patients. • Developing multidisciplinary implementation teams that bring together experts in different approaches. • Applying insights derived from other disciplines to solve healthcare issues. • Positioning new empirical investigations against previous relevant studies and building on, rather than reinventing, previous knowledge.
Integration of knowledge about determinants, mechanisms, and outcomes of implementation	• Increasing the use of longitudinal designs to uncover the emergent properties of implementation and its delayed consequences. • Focusing data analysis on developing themes that link different elements of the causal pathway together. • Linking the findings of process and outcome evaluations of the same intervention. • Complementing existing determinant frameworks with novel approaches to identify mechanisms of implementation and capture its outcomes (including economic evaluations).

Crossing the boundaries between researchers, practitioners, and service users

- Producing how-to guides on implementation with and for practitioners.
- Developing and evaluating participatory approaches to implementation, particularly those involving co-production with service users.
- Developing new approaches for achieving an adequate match between a practical issue and a scientific approach used to address it.
- Moving away from tightly controlling interventions to more flexible designs that enable feedback loops with all implementation stakeholders.

7 Further Reading

Much of the literature cited in this Element is freely and permanently accessible online without subscription charges or registration barriers. The following resources represent in our view the best introductory primers for those interested in more in-depth learning about the field.

- Brownson et al.[116] – an introductory text for researchers and practitioners focused on key concepts and critical elements in research design and evaluation.
- National Cancer Institute[117] – a workbook written by members of the institute's implementation science team. It outlines key theories, methods, and models and serves as a guide to how implementation science can support the adoption of evidence-based interventions.
- Wensing et al.[118] – an introductory text for practitioners and policy-makers providing an evidence-based and practical model for implementing practice change and innovation.

Contributors

Paul Wilson and Roman Kislov conceived the Element. Paul Wilson drafted the initial manuscript with the exception of Section 5, which was drafted by Roman Kislov. Both authors contributed equally to subsequent drafts and have approved the final version.

Conflicts of Interest

Paul Wilson is Co-Editor-in-Chief of the journal *Implementation Science* and Roman Kislov is Associate Editor of the journal *Implementation Science Communications*. Paul Wilson and Roman Kislov are in receipt of funding from the National Institute for Health Research (NIHR) Applied Research Collaboration Greater Manchester. The views expressed in this Element are those of the authors and not necessarily those of the NHS, NIHR, or Department of Health and Social Care.

Acknowledgements

We thank the peer reviewers and editors for their insightful comments and recommendations to improve the Element. A list of peer reviewers is published at www.cambridge.org/IQ-peer-reviewers.

Funding

This Element was funded by THIS Institute (The Healthcare Improvement Studies Institute, www.thisinstitute.cam.ac.uk). THIS Institute is strengthening the evidence base for improving the quality and safety of healthcare. THIS Institute is supported by a grant to the University of Cambridge from the Health Foundation – an independent charity committed to bringing about better health and healthcare for people in the UK.

About the Authors

Paul Wilson is a senior lecturer at the University of Manchester, Theme Lead on Implementation Science for the NIHR Applied Research Collaboration Greater Manchester, and Co-Editor-in-Chief of *Implementation Science*. His research interests focus on the role and use of evidence to inform decisions relating to service delivery, redesign, and disinvestment.

Roman Kislov is a professor of health policy and management at Manchester Metropolitan University, and Deputy Theme Lead on Implementation Science for the NIHR Applied Research Collaboration Greater Manchester. He conducts qualitative research on the processes and practices of knowledge mobilisation.

Creative Commons Licence

References

1. Eccles MP, Mittman BS. Welcome to implementation science. *Implement Sci* 2006; 1: 1. https://doi.org/10.1186/1748-5908-1-1.

2. Proctor E, Silmere H, Raghavan R, et al. Outcomes for implementation research: conceptual distinctions, measurement challenges, and research agenda. *Adm Policy Ment Health* 2011; 38: 65–76. https://doi.org/10.1007/s10488-010-0319-7.

3. Prasad V, Ioannidis JP. Evidence-based de-implementation for contradicted, unproven, and aspiring healthcare practices. *Implement Sci* 2014; 9: 1. https://doi.org/10.1186/1748-5908-9-1.

4. Norton WE, Chambers DA. Unpacking the complexities of de-implementing inappropriate health interventions. *Implement Sci* 2020; 15: 2. https://doi.org/10.1186/s13012-019-0960-9.

5. Craig P, Dieppe P, Macintyre S, et al. Developing and evaluating complex interventions: the new Medical Research Council guidance. *BMJ* 2008; 337: a1655. https://doi.org/10.1136/bmj.a1655.

6. Moore GF, Audrey S, Barker M, et al. Process evaluation of complex interventions: Medical Research Council guidance. *BMJ* 2015; 350: h1258. https://doi.org/10.1136/bmj.h1258.

7. Roberts MC, Kennedy AE, Chambers DA, Khoury MJ. The current state of implementation science in genomic medicine: opportunities for improvement. *Genet Med* 2017; 19: 858–63. https://doi.org/10.1038/gim.2016.210.

8. Patey AM, Hurt CS, Grimshaw JM, Francis JJ. Changing behaviour 'more or less' – do theories of behaviour inform strategies for implementation and de-implementation? A critical interpretive synthesis. *Implement Sci* 2018; 13: 134. https://doi.org/10.1186/s13012-018-0826-6.

9. van Bodegom-Vos L, Davidoff F, Marang-van de Mheen PJ. Implementation and de-implementation: two sides of the same coin? *BMJ Qual Saf* 2017; 26: 495–501. https://doi.org/10.1136/bmjqs-2016-005473.

10. Norton WE, Chambers DA, Kramer BS. Conceptualizing de-implementation in cancer care delivery. *J Clin Oncol* 2019; 37: 93–6. https://doi.org/10.1200/jco.18.00589.

11. Grimshaw JM, Patey AM, Kirkham KR, et al. De-implementing wisely: developing the evidence base to reduce low-value care. *BMJ Qual Saf* 2020; 29: 409. https://doi.org/10.1136/bmjqs-2019-010060.

12. Spiegelhalter DJ. Surgical audit: statistical lessons from Nightingale and Codman. *J Roy Stat Soc Ser A (Stat Soc)* 1999; 162: 45–58. https://doi.org/10.1111/1467-985X.00120.

13. Codman EA. The classic: a study in hospital efficiency: as demonstrated by the case report of first five years of private hospital. *Clin Orthop Relat Res* 2013; 471: 1778–83. https://doi.org/10.1007/s11999-012-2751-3.

14. Glover JA. The incidence of tonsillectomy in school children: (Section of Epidemiology and State Medicine). *Pro R Soc Medicine* 1938; 31: 1219–36. https://pubmed.ncbi.nlm.nih.gov/19991659 (accessed 8 April 2022).

15. Donabedian A. Evaluating the quality of medical care. *Milbank Q* 2005 (reprinted from 1966); 83: 691–729. https://doi.org/10.1111/j.1468-0009.2005.00397.x.

16. Lembcke PA. Medical auditing by scientific methods: illustrated by major female pelvic surgery. *JAMA* 1956; 162: 646–55. https://doi.org/10.1001/jama.1956.72970240010009.

17. Mitchell MW, Fowkes FG. Audit reviewed: does feedback on performance change clinical behaviour? *J R Coll Physicians Lond* 1985; 19: 251–4. https://pubmed.ncbi.nlm.nih.gov/4067901 (accessed 8 April 2022).

18. Grol R, Mokkink H, Schellevis F. The effects of peer review in general practice. *J R Coll Gen Pract* 1988; 38: 10–3. https://pubmed.ncbi.nlm.nih.gov/3204541 (accessed 8 April 2022).

19. Ivers N, Jamtvedt G, Flottorp S, et al. Audit and feedback: effects on professional practice and healthcare outcomes. *Cochrane Database Syst Rev* 2012; 6: CD000259. https://doi.org/10.1002/14651858.CD000259.pub3.

20. Ivers N, Foy R. Audit, feedback, and behaviour change. In: Dixon-Woods M, Brown K, Marjanovic S, et al., editors. *Elements of Improving Quality and Safety in Healthcare*. Cambridge: Cambridge University Press; forthcoming.

21. Rogers EM. *Diffusion of Innovations, 5th ed*. London: Free Press; 2003.

22. Greenhalgh T, Robert G, Bate P, Macfarlane F, Kyriakidou O. *Diffusion of Innovations in Health Service Organisations: A Systematic Literature Review*. Oxford: Blackwell; 2005. https://doi.org/10.1002/9780470987407.

23. Coleman J, Katz E, Menzel H. The diffusion of an innovation among physicians. *Sociometry* 1957; 20: 253–70. https://doi.org/10.2307/2785979.

24. Brook RH, Chassin MR, Fink A, et al. A method for the detailed assessment of the appropriateness of medical technologies. *Int J Technol Assess Health Care* 1986; 2: 53–63. https://doi.org/10.1017/s0266462300002774.

25. Woolf SH, Agency for Health Care Policy and Research. *Interim Manual for Clinical Practice Guideline Development*. Agency for Health Care Policy and Research, US Department of Health and Human Services, Public Health Service; 1991.

26. Lomas J, Anderson GM, Domnick-Pierre K, et al. Do practice guidelines guide practice? The effect of a consensus statement on the practice of physicians. *N Engl J Med* 1989; 321: 1306–11. https://doi.org/10.1056/nejm198911093211906.

27. Lomas J. Diffusion, dissemination, and implementation: who should do what? *Ann N Y Acad Sci* 1993; 703: 226–35; discussion 235–7. https://doi.org/10.1111/j.1749-6632.1993.tb26351.x.

28. Soumerai SB, McLaughlin TJ, Avorn J. Improving drug prescribing in primary care: a critical analysis of the experimental literature. *Milbank Q* 1989; 67: 268–317. https://pubmed.ncbi.nlm.nih.gov/2698446 (accessed 8 April 2022).

29. Grol R. Implementing guidelines in general practice care. *Qual Health Care* 1992; 1: 184–91. https://doi.org/10.1136/qshc.1.3.184.

30. Grimshaw JM, Russell IT. Effect of clinical guidelines on medical practice: a systematic review of rigorous evaluations. *Lancet* 1993; 342: 1317–22. https://doi.org/10.1016/0140-6736(93)92244-n.

31. Sechrest L, Backer TE, Rogers EM, Campbell TF, Grady ML. *Effective Dissemination of Clinical Health Information: Conference Summary*. Rockville, MD: Agency for Health Care Policy and Research; 1994. AHCPR report no. 95-0015.

32. NHS Centre for Reviews and Dissemination. Implementing clinical practice guidelines: can guidelines be used to improve clinical practice? *Eff Health Care* 1994; 8. www.york.ac.uk/media/crd/ehc18.pdf (accessed 8 April 2022).

33. NHS Centre for Reviews and Dissemination. Getting evidence into practice. *Eff Health Care* 1999; 5: 1. www.york.ac.uk/media/crd/ehc51.pdf (accessed 8 April 2022).

34. Michie S, Johnston M. Changing clinical behaviour by making guidelines specific. *BMJ* 2004; 328: 343–5. https://doi.org/10.1136/bmj.328.7435.343.

35. Straus SE, Brouwers M, Johnson D, et al. Core competencies in the science and practice of knowledge translation: description of a Canadian strategic training initiative. *Implement Sci* 2011; 6: 127. https://doi.org/10.1186/1748-5908-6-127.

36. Proctor EK, Chambers DA. Training in dissemination and implementation research: a field-wide perspective. *Transl Behav Med* 2017; 7: 624–35. https://doi.org/10.1007/s13142-016-0406-8.

37. Stetler CB, Mittman BS, Francis J. Overview of the VA quality enhancement research initiative (QUERI) and QUERI theme articles: QUERI series. *Implement Sci* 2008; 3: 8. https://doi.org/10.1186/1748-5908-3-8.

38. Atkins D, Kilbourne AM, Shulkin D. Moving from discovery to system-wide change: the role of research in a learning health care system: experience from three decades of health systems research in the Veterans Health Administration. *Annu Rev Public Health* 2017; 38: 467–87. https://doi.org/10.1146/annurev-publhealth-031816-044255.

39. Kislov R, Wilson PM, Knowles S, Boaden R. Learning from the emergence of NIHR Collaborations for Leadership in Applied Health Research and Care (CLAHRCs): a systematic review of evaluations. *Implement Sci* 2018; 13: 111. https://doi.org/10.1186/s13012-018-0805-y.

40. Presseau J, McCleary N, Lorencatto F, et al. Action, actor, context, target, time (AACTT): a framework for specifying behaviour. *Implement Sci* 2019; 14: 102. https://doi.org/10.1186/s13012-019-0951-x.

41. Ross J, Stevenson F, Lau R, Murray E. Factors that influence the implementation of e-health: a systematic review of systematic reviews (an update). *Implement Sci* 2016; 11: 146. https://doi.org/10.1186/s13012-016-0510-7.

42. Cochrane Effective Practice and Organisation of Care (EPOC). *EPOC taxonomy* 2015. https://epoc.cochrane.org/epoc-taxonomy (accessed 8 April 2022).

43. Proctor EK, Powell BJ, McMillen JC. Implementation strategies: recommendations for specifying and reporting. *Implement Sci* 2013; 8: 139. https://doi.org/10.1186/1748-5908-8-139.

44. Brehaut JC, Colquhoun HL, Eva KW, et al. Practice feedback interventions: 15 suggestions for optimizing effectiveness. *Ann Intern Med* 2016; 164: 435–41. https://doi.org/10.7326/m15-2248.

45. Shojania KG, Jennings A, Mayhew A, et al. The effects of on-screen, point of care computer reminders on processes and outcomes of care. *Cochrane Database Syst Rev* 2009; 3: CD001096. https://doi.org/10.1002/14651858 .CD001096.pub2.

46. Kwan JL, Lo L, Ferguson J, et al. Computerised clinical decision support systems and absolute improvements in care: meta-analysis of controlled clinical trials. *BMJ* 2020; 370: m3216. https://doi.org/10.1136/bmj .m3216.

47. Forsetlund L, Bjørndal A, Rashidian A, et al. Continuing education meetings and workshops: effects on professional practice and health care outcomes. *Cochrane Database Syst Rev* 2009; 2: CD003030. https://doi .org/10.1002/14651858.CD003030.pub2.

48. O'Brien MA, Rogers S, Jamtvedt G, et al. Educational outreach visits: effects on professional practice and health care outcomes. *Cochrane Database Syst Rev* 2007; 4: CD000409. https://doi.org/10.1002/14651858.CD000409.pub2.

49. Harvey G, Kitson A. PARIHS revisited: from heuristic to integrated framework for the successful implementation of knowledge into practice. *Implement Sci* 2016; 11: 33. https://doi.org/10.1186/s13012-016-0398-2.

50. Cranley LA, Cummings GG, Profetto-McGrath J, Toth F, Estabrooks CA. Facilitation roles and characteristics associated with research use by healthcare professionals: a scoping review. *BMJ Open* 2017; 7: e014384. https://doi.org/10.1136/bmjopen-2016-014384.

51. Flodgren G, Eccles MP, Shepperd S, et al. An overview of reviews evaluating the effectiveness of financial incentives in changing healthcare professional behaviours and patient outcomes. *Cochrane Database Syst Rev* 2011; 7: CD009255. https://doi.org/10.1002/14651858.CD009255.

52. Mendelson A, Kondo K, Damberg C, et al. The effects of pay-for-performance programs on health, health care use, and processes of care: a systematic review. *Ann Intern Med* 2017; 166: 341–53. https://doi.org/10.7326/m16-1881.

53. Flodgren G, O'Brien MA, Parmelli E, Grimshaw JM. Local opinion leaders: effects on professional practice and healthcare outcomes. *Cochrane Database Syst Rev* 2019; 6: CD000125. https://doi.org/10.1002/14651858.CD000125.pub5.

54. Giguère A, Zomahoun HTV, Carmichael PH, et al. Printed educational materials: effects on professional practice and healthcare outcomes. *Cochrane Database Syst Rev* 2020; 8: CD004398. https://doi.org/10.1002/14651858.CD004398.pub4.

55. Hulscher ME, Schouten LM, Grol RP, Buchan H. Determinants of success of quality improvement collaboratives: what does the literature show? *BMJ Qual Saf* 2013; 22: 19–31. https://doi.org/10.1136/bmjqs-2011-000651.

56. Wells S, Tamir O, Gray J, et al. Are quality improvement collaboratives effective? A systematic review. *BMJ Qual Saf* 2018; 27: 226–40. https://doi.org/10.1136/bmjqs-2017-006926.

57. Powell BJ, Waltz TJ, Chinman MJ, et al. A refined compilation of implementation strategies: results from the Expert Recommendations for Implementing Change (ERIC) project. *Implement Sci* 2015; 10: 21. https://doi.org/10.1186/s13012-015-0209-1.

58. Wensing M, Grol R. Single and combined strategies for implementing changes in primary care: a literature review. *Int J Qual Health Care* 1994; 6: 115–32. https://doi.org/10.1093/intqhc/6.2.115.

59. Oxman AD, Thomson MA, Davis DA, Haynes RB. No magic bullets: a systematic review of 102 trials of interventions to improve professional practice. *CMAJ* 1995; 153: 1423–31. https://pubmed.ncbi.nlm.nih.gov/7585368/ (accessed 8 April 2022).

60. Ivers NM, Grimshaw JM, Jamtvedt G, et al. Growing literature, stagnant science? Systematic review, meta-regression and cumulative analysis of audit and feedback interventions in health care. *J Gen Intern Med* 2014; 29: 1534–41. https://doi.org/10.1007/s11606-014-2913-y.

61. Lewis CC, Boyd MR, Walsh-Bailey C, et al. A systematic review of empirical studies examining mechanisms of implementation in health. *Implement Sci* 2020; 15: 21. https://doi.org/10.1186/s13012-020-00983-3.

62. Wensing M. The tailored implementation in chronic diseases (TICD) project: introduction and main findings. *Implement Sci* 2017; 12: 5. https://doi.org/10.1186/s13012-016-0536-x.

63. Grimshaw JM, Ivers N, Linklater S, et al. Reinvigorating stagnant science: implementation laboratories and a meta-laboratory to efficiently advance the science of audit and feedback. *BMJ Qual Saf* 2019; 28: 416–23. https://doi.org/10.1136/bmjqs-2018-008355.

64. Powell BJ, Fernandez ME, Williams NJ, et al. Enhancing the impact of implementation strategies in healthcare: a research agenda. *Front Public Health* 2019; 7: 3. https://doi.org/10.3389/fpubh.2019.00003.

65. Avery AJ, Rodgers S, Cantrill JA, et al. A pharmacist-led information technology intervention for medication errors (PINCER): a multicentre, cluster randomised, controlled trial and cost-effectiveness analysis. *Lancet* 2012; 379: 1310–19. https://doi.org/10.1016/s0140-6736(11)61817-5.

66. Grimshaw JM, Thomas RE, MacLennan G, et al. Effectiveness and efficiency of guideline dissemination and implementation strategies. *Health Technol Assess* 2004; 8: 6. https://doi.org/10.3310/hta8060.

67. Hawe P, Shiell A, Riley T. Theorising interventions as events in systems. *Am J Community Psychol* 2009; 43: 267–76. https://doi.org/10.1007/s10464-009-9229-9.

68. May CR, Johnson M, Finch T. Implementation, context and complexity. *Implement Sci* 2016; 11: 141. https://doi.org/10.1186/s13012-016-0506-3.

69. Tabak RG, Khoong EC, Chambers DA, Brownson RC. Bridging research and practice: models for dissemination and implementation research. *Am J Prev Med* 2012; 43: 337–50. https://doi.org/10.1016/j.amepre.2012.05.024.

70. Nilsen P. Making sense of implementation theories, models and frameworks. *Implement Sci* 2015; 10: 53. https://doi.org/10.1186/s13012-015-0242-0.

71. Damschroder LJ, Aron DC, Keith RE, et al. Fostering implementation of health services research findings into practice: a consolidated framework for advancing implementation science. *Implement Sci* 2009; 4: 50. https://doi.org/10.1186/1748-5908-4-50.

72. Kirk MA, Kelley C, Yankey N, et al. A systematic review of the use of the consolidated framework for implementation research. *Implement Sci* 2016; 11: 72. https://doi.org/10.1186/s13012-016-0437-z.

73. Michie S, van Stralen MM, West R. The behaviour change wheel: a new method for characterising and designing behaviour change interventions. *Implement Sci* 2011; 6: 42. https://doi.org/10.1186/1748-5908-6-42.

74. Kitson A, Harvey G, McCormack B. Enabling the implementation of evidence based practice: a conceptual framework. *Qual Health Care* 1998; 7: 149–58. https://doi.org/10.1136/qshc.7.3.149.

75. Helfrich CD, Damschroder LJ, Hagedorn HJ, et al. A critical synthesis of literature on the promoting action on research implementation in health services (PARIHS) framework. *Implement Sci* 2010; 5: 82. https://doi.org/10.1186/1748-5908-5-82.

76. May CR, Mair F, Finch T, et al. Development of a theory of implementation and integration: Normalization Process Theory. *Implement Sci* 2009; 4: 29. https://doi.org/10.1186/1748-5908-4-29.

77. May CR, Cummings A, Girling M, et al. Using Normalization Process Theory in feasibility studies and process evaluations of complex healthcare interventions: a systematic review. *Implement Sci* 2018; 13: 80. https://doi.org/10.1186/s13012-018-0758-1.

78. Glasgow RE, Vogt TM, Boles SM. Evaluating the public health impact of health promotion interventions: the RE-AIM framework. *Am J Public Health* 1999; 89: 1322–7. https://doi.org/10.2105/ajph.89.9.1322.

79. Glasgow RE, Harden SM, Gaglio B, et al. RE-AIM planning and evaluation framework: adapting to new science and practice with a 20-year review. *Front Publ Health* 2019; 7: 64. https://doi.org/10.3389/fpubh.2019.00064.

80. Cane J, O'Connor D, Michie S. Validation of the theoretical domains framework for use in behaviour change and implementation research. *Implement Sci* 2012; 7: 37. https://doi.org/10.1186/1748-5908-7-37.

81. Atkins L, Francis J, Islam R, et al. A guide to using the Theoretical Domains Framework of behaviour change to investigate implementation

problems. *Implement Sci* 2017; 12: 77. https://doi.org/10.1186/s13012-017-0605-9.

82. Michie S, Johnston M, Abraham C, et al. Making psychological theory useful for implementing evidence based practice: a consensus approach. *Qual Saf Health Care* 2005; 14: 26–33. https://doi.org/10.1136/qshc.2004.011155.

83. Moore JE, Rashid S, Park JS, Khan S, Straus SE. Longitudinal evaluation of a course to build core competencies in implementation practice. *Implement Sci* 2018; 13: 106. https://doi.org/10.1186/s13012-018-0800-3.

84. Birken SA, Rohweder CL, Powell BJ, et al. T-CaST: an implementation theory comparison and selection tool. *Implement Sci* 2018; 13: 143. https://doi.org/10.1186/s13012-018-0836-4.

85. Lynch EA, Mudge A, Knowles S, et al. 'There is nothing so practical as a good theory': a pragmatic guide for selecting theoretical approaches for implementation projects. *BMC Health Serv Res* 2018; 18: 857. https://doi.org/10.1186/s12913-018-3671-z.

86. Strifler L, Barnsley JM, Hillmer M, Straus SE. Identifying and selecting implementation theories, models and frameworks: a qualitative study to inform the development of a decision support tool. *BMC Med Inform Decis Mak* 2020; 20: 91. https://doi.org/10.1186/s12911-020-01128-8.

87. Moullin JC, Dickson KS, Stadnick NA, et al. Ten recommendations for using implementation frameworks in research and practice. *Implement Sci Commun* 2020; 1: 42. https://doi.org/10.1186/s43058-020-00023-7.

88. Foley T, Horwitz L. Learning health systems. In: Dixon-Woods M, Brown K, Marjanovic S, et al., editors. *Elements of Improving Quality and Safety in Healthcare*. Cambridge: Cambridge University Press; forthcoming.

89. US Department of Veterans Affairs. QUERI – Quality Enhancement Research Initiative. www.queri.research.va.gov/default.cfm (accessed 8 April 2022).

90. Stetler CB, Mittman BS, Francis J, Eccles M, Graham ID, editors. US Department of Veterans Affairs Quality Enhancement Research Initiative (QUERI). *Implement Sci* 2008–09. www.biomedcentral.com/collections/1748-5908-Que (accessed 8 April 2022).

91. O'Hanlon C, Huang C, Sloss E, et al. Comparing VA and non-VA quality of care: a systematic review. *J Gen Intern Med* 2017; 32: 105–21. https://doi.org/10.1007/s11606-016-3775-2.

92. Braganza MZ, Kilbourne AM. The quality enhancement research initiative (QUERI) impact framework: measuring the real-world impact of implementation science. *J Gen Intern Med* 2021; 36: 396–403. https://doi.org/10.1007/s11606-020-06143-z.

93. Boulton R, Sandall J, Sevdalis N. The cultural politics of 'implementation science'. *J Med Humanit* 2020; 41: 379–94. https://doi.org/10.1007/s10912-020-09607-9.

94. Wensing M, Grol R. Knowledge translation in health: how implementation science could contribute more. *BMC Med* 2019; 17: 88. https://doi.org/10.1186/s12916-019-1322-9.

95. Kislov R, Pope C, Martin GP, Wilson PM. Harnessing the power of theorising in implementation science. *Implement Sci* 2019; 14: 103. https://doi.org/10.1186/s13012-019-0957-4.

96. Patton MQ. *Qualitative Research & Evaluation Methods: Integrating Theory and Practice, 4th ed.* Thousand Oaks, CA: Sage; 2015.

97. Lewis CC, Klasnja P, Powell BJ, et al. From classification to causality: advancing understanding of mechanisms of change in implementation science. *Front Public Health* 2018; 6: 136. https://doi.org/10.3389/fpubh.2018.00136.

98. Graham ID, Logan J, Harrison MB, et al. Lost in knowledge translation: time for a map? *J Contin Educ Health Prof* 2006; 26: 13–24. https://doi.org/10.1002/chp.47.

99. Hedström P, Ylikoski P. Causal mechanisms in the social sciences. *Annu Rev Sociol* 2010; 36: 49–67. https://doi.org/10.1146/annurev.soc.012809.102632.

100. Berta W, Cranley L, Dearing JW, et al. Why (we think) facilitation works: insights from organizational learning theory. *Implement Sci* 2015; 10: 141. https://doi.org/10.1186/s13012-015-0323-0.

101. Kislov R, Humphreys J, Harvey G. How do managerial techniques evolve over time? The distortion of 'facilitation' in healthcare service improvement. *Publ Manage Rev* 2017; 19: 1165–83. https://doi.org/10.1080/14719037.2016.1266022.

102. Seers K, Rycroft-Malone J, Cox K, et al. Facilitating implementation of research evidence (FIRE): an international cluster randomised controlled trial to evaluate two models of facilitation informed by the promoting action on research implementation in health services (PARIHS) framework. *Implement Sci* 2018; 13: 137. https://doi.org/10.1186/s13012-018-0831-9.

103. Rycroft-Malone J, Seers K, Eldh AC, et al. A realist process evaluation within the Facilitating Implementation of Research Evidence (FIRE) cluster randomised controlled international trial: an exemplar. *Implement Sci* 2018; 13: 138. https://doi.org/10.1186/s13012-018-0811-0.

104. Harvey G, McCormack B, Kitson A, Lynch E, Titchen A. Designing and implementing two facilitation interventions within the 'Facilitating

Implementation of Research Evidence (FIRE)' study: a qualitative analysis from an external facilitators' perspective. *Implement Sci* 2018; 13: 141. https://doi.org/10.1186/s13012-018-0812-z.

105. Dickinson H, Sullivan H. Towards a general theory of collaborative performance: the importance of efficacy and agency. *Public Admin* 2014; 92: 161–77. https://doi.org/10.1111/padm.12048.

106. Hoomans T, Severens JL. Economic evaluation of implementation strategies in health care. *Implement Sci* 2014; 9: 168. https://doi.org/10.1186/s13012-014-0168-y.

107. Street A, Gutacker N. Health economics. In: Dixon-Woods M, Brown K, Marjanovic S, et al., editors. *Elements of Improving Quality and Safety in Healthcare*. Cambridge: Cambridge University Press; forthcoming.

108. Vale L, Thomas R, MacLennan G, Grimshaw J. Systematic review of economic evaluations and cost analyses of guideline implementation strategies. *Eur J Health Econ* 2007; 8: 111–21. https://doi.org/10.1007/s10198-007-0043-8.

109. Roberts SLE, Healey A, Sevdalis N. Use of health economic evaluation in the implementation and improvement science fields-a systematic literature review. *Implement Sci* 2019; 14: 72. https://doi.org/10.1186/s13012-019-0901-7.

110. Walshe K. Pseudoinnovation: the development and spread of healthcare quality improvement methodologies. *Int J Qual Health Care* 2009; 21: 153–9. https://doi.org/10.1093/intqhc/mzp012.

111. De Silva MJ, Breuer E, Lee L, et al. Theory of change: a theory-driven approach to enhance the Medical Research Council's framework for complex interventions. *Trials* 2014; 15: 267. https://doi.org/10.1186/1745-6215-15-267.

112. Ivers NM, Grimshaw JM. Reducing research waste with implementation laboratories. *Lancet* 2016; 388: 547–8. https://doi.org/10.1016/s0140-6736(16)31256-9.

113. Reed JE, Howe C, Doyle C, Bell D. Simple rules for evidence translation in complex systems: a qualitative study. *BMC Med* 2018; 16: 92. https://doi.org/10.1186/s12916-018-1076-9.

114. O'Hara JK, Aase K, Waring J. Scaffolding our systems? Patients and families 'reaching in' as a source of healthcare resilience. *BMJ Qual Saf* 2019; 28: 3–6. https://doi.org/10.1136/bmjqs-2018-008216.

115. Robert G, Locock L, Williams O, et al. Co-producing and co-designing. In: Dixon-Woods M, Brown K, Marjanovic S, et al., editors. *Elements of Improving Quality and Safety in Healthcare*. Cambridge:

Cambridge University Press; 2022. https://doi.org/10.1017/9781009 237024.

116. Brownson RC, Colditz GA, Proctor EK, editors. *Dissemination and Implementation Research in Health: Translating Science to Practice, 2nd ed.* Oxford: Oxford University Press; 2018. https://doi.org/10.1093/acprof:oso/9780199751877.001.0001.

117. National Cancer Institute. *Implementation Science at a Glance: A Guide for Cancer Control Practitioners*. US Department of Health and Human Services, National Institutes of Health. https://cancercontrol.cancer.gov/is/tools/practice-tools (accessed 8 April 2022).

118. Wensing M, Grol R, Grimshaw J, editors. *Improving Patient Care: The Implementation of Change in Health Care, 3rd ed.* Chichester: John Wiley & Sons; 2020. https://doi.org/10.1002/9781119488620.

Cambridge Elements ☰

Improving Quality and Safety in Healthcare

Editors-in-Chief

Mary Dixon-Woods
THIS Institute (The Healthcare Improvement Studies Institute)

Mary is Director of THIS Institute and is the Health Foundation Professor of Healthcare Improvement Studies in the Department of Public Health and Primary Care at the University of Cambridge. Mary leads a programme of research focused on healthcare improvement, healthcare ethics, and methodological innovation in studying healthcare.

Graham Martin
THIS Institute (The Healthcare Improvement Studies Institute)

Graham is Director of Research at THIS Institute, leading applied research programmes and contributing to the institute's strategy and development. His research interests are in the organisation and delivery of healthcare, and particularly the role of professionals, managers, and patients and the public in efforts at organisational change.

Executive Editor

Katrina Brown
THIS Institute (The Healthcare Improvement Studies Institute)

Katrina is Communications Manager at THIS Institute, providing editorial expertise to maximise the impact of THIS Institute's research findings. She managed the project to produce the series.

Editorial Team

Sonja Marjanovic
RAND Europe

Sonja is Director of RAND Europe's healthcare innovation, industry, and policy research. Her work provides decision-makers with evidence and insights to support innovation and improvement in healthcare systems, and to support the translation of innovation into societal benefits for healthcare services and population health.

Tom Ling
RAND Europe

Tom is Head of Evaluation at RAND Europe and President of the European Evaluation Society, leading evaluations and applied research focused on the key challenges facing health services. His current health portfolio includes evaluations of the innovation landscape, quality improvement, communities of practice, patient flow, and service transformation.

Ellen Perry
THIS Institute (The Healthcare Improvement Studies Institute)
Ellen supported the production of the series during 2020–21.

About the Series

The past decade has seen enormous growth in both activity and research on improvement in healthcare. This series offers a comprehensive and authoritative set of overviews of the different improvement approaches available, exploring the thinking behind them, examining evidence for each approach, and identifying areas of debate.

Cambridge Elements $\equiv$

Improving Quality and Safety in Healthcare

Elements in the Series

Collaboration-Based Approaches
Graham Martin and Mary Dixon-Woods

Co-Producing and Co-Designing
Glenn Robert, Louise Locock, Oli Williams, Jocelyn Cornwell, Sara Donetto, and
Joanna Goodrich

The Positive Deviance Approach
Ruth Baxter and Rebecca Lawton

Implementation Science
Paul Wilson and Roman Kislov

Making Culture Change Happen
Russell Mannion

Operational Research Approaches
Martin Utley, Sonya Crowe, and Christina Pagel

A full series listing is available at: www.cambridge.org/IQ